Simple Ways to Improve Blood Circulation

The Benefits of Improving Blood Circulation for a Healthy Life

Message from the Author

I believe in bringing happiness to people and help the people in needed is the purpose of my life. One of the ways is to share the knowledge that I know to the people. Time is the most valuable thing. You only live once, so you should make the most of it, just enjoy your life with no regrets. Even if you have money, you cannot do anything if you do not have a healthy body. Publishing this book life fulfilling and it means a lot to me. Thank you for your support, if you encounter any kinds of health problems, don't run away as it will come to you eventually. Face it with courage, be positive and have a happy mindset, believe that our body can fight off any disease if we find the right method and fight it persistently. Never go down without a fight. I hope this book can help you to live a healthy life!

Alan To

1

Table of Contents

The Importance of Proper Blood Circulation

Every human body is coursing with the serum of life; Blood. Without it, essentially none of our bodily functions or organs would work. Without it, we would not exist.

Blood consists of three parts; Plasma, red blood cells, and clotting agents. Together they make whole blood. Whole blood delivers vital nutrients, oxygen, hormones, and sugars to our cells. Blood also performs another important duty of carrying away waste from our cells, which is expelled from our body through our urine, excrement, sweat glands, and through our breath when we exhale.

Blood plays an important role in how our bodies look, function, and heal. If you have ever had a wound you might recall that the area would become red and swollen. That is because the circulation of blood to that area has been increased, prompted by the perception of pain by the brain. Signals from your brain are sent to your body with instructions to do damage control and begin to heal the area through a very complex process. Increased blood flow to an area of injury delivers white blood cells to fight off infection, platelets that stick together to prevent blood loss, and collagen to begin growing new skin.

Simple Ways to Improve Blood Circulation

A famous English physician, William Harvey (1578-1657), discovered that the systemic circulation and properties of blood being pumped to the body and brain by heart, and the blood circulation of our bodies keep us alive. So just imagine, if the blood cannot circulate smoothly within our bodies, how we can have a body that functions properly and live a healthy life.

In the Bible, it mentions that the blood is the life.

Only be sure that thou eat not the *blood*: for the *blood is* the *life*; and thou mayest not eat the *life* with the flesh.
Deuteronomy 12:23

For it *is* the *life* of all flesh; the *blood* of it *is* for the *life* thereof:
Leviticus 17:14

If the blood is not flowing within us, no energy will flow within us. Therefore loss too much blood will endanger our lives. On the same hand, if someone has some problem with their heart beat, we have to perform Cardiopulmonary resuscitation (CPR) to restore spontaneous blood circulation and breathing in a person who is in cardiac arrest immediately. Even though CPR does not restart the heart, it can restore partial flow of oxygenated blood to the brain and heart. If the blood circulation stops for

4 minutes or above, there is a chance that the brain can be damaged permanently due to lack of oxygen.

Adequate blood circulation dictates what kind of appearance we have, which could affect opportunities in life such as job opportunities, promotions, finding partners, and even how you are treated by the general public. Poor blood circulation also impacts multiple metabolic and cardiovascular functions throughout your whole body.

In Winter, water in the river is frozen which does not flow, if we generate heat into the river, then water will flow, if we generate higher temperature into the river, water will vapor and transform to the cloud in the sky. In Chinese, the energy that transforms water from liquid to gas is called "Chi". Only the living creatures have "Chi", "Chi" can keep you breathing, no one can live without "Chi".

The following chapters will take you through the various ways proper blood circulation plays a crucial role in your life, and why it is important to maintain your cardiovascular system for proper blood circulation.

The Benefits of Proper Blood Circulation

Good circulation plays a large part in our appearance. It is programmed into our DNA to recognize a person with good color to their face and body (think rosy cheeks), as an indicator of good health. Appearance is everything. You have heard it before, and it will continue to be a part of our cultural ways of gauging social status, acceptance, who will be our leaders, who we will reproduce with, spend time with, work with, and even provide aid to.

You will be able to reap the rewards of a more youthful look throughout your entire life if you maintain proper blood circulation. People who exercise regularly, and do not smoke, maintain a healthier, youthful look well into their later years. Usually, healthy people are more attractive than unhealthy people, as the appearance is a strong indicator for a person's health. Remember this rule, "All beautiful people are healthy". No one can be beautiful but live a unhealthy life. Healthy complexions tell us that the person is probably well fed, and of a good social status. It is a harsh reality that so much is dependent on our appearance.

Sufficient blood circulation has a profound impact on our bodies appearance and function as a whole. The ability to enjoy a good

6

quality of life with less illness, perform and enjoy physical exercise, and a youthful vibrant appearance, rests solely on proper circulation. Some people looks very old at the age of 30, while some people looks very young at the age of 40 or even 50. The difference is that the people who have youthful appearance live a healthy life and proper blood circulation is a must.

The blood in our bodies plays an important role in our immune systems and our ability to fight off infections, even before we show any signs or symptoms of an invasion. Blood delivers T and B lymphocytes through our blood stream, releasing antibodies that attack intrusive bodies as well as "tag" them so the other blood cells can identify and destroy them.

A strong immune system is essential in order to support quality of life. Proper blood circulation can help reduce the incidence of upper respiratory tract infections (URTI). Maintaining healthy circulation throughout your life can help you avoid aging, memory loss, strokes, heart attacks, a decrease in kidney function, and undesirable changes in skin tone.

Adequate blood circulation also prevents pain caused by poor circulation. This could be a pain in the lower extremities, and general muscle soreness that many people mistake for over-exertion or a pulled muscle. In fact, the pain they are experiencing is due to poor circulation. Proper blood circulation can remove substances that were clogging in your blood stream. We feel pain or itchy sometimes is because of toxic substances are existing under our skin.

Maintaining healthy levels of blood circulation has a very crucial role in sustaining proper brain function. Clarity of thought and an excellent memory are just a couple of the benefits of healthy circulation and adequate oxygen delivery to your brain, which alone uses about 20% of the total oxygen in our bodies. In some extreme situations, blood clots in the brain may leads to amnesia.

Proper blood circulation reaches into all aspects of our lives and the way we are able to enjoy it. This includes having enough energy to engage in the tasks and activities we love and enjoy. From working out at the gym to swimming in the lake, spending a day at the fair with your family, or having a satisfying sex life with our love one. Healthy people also earn more money in their lifetime because they spend more time at work, not having to take as many sick days off. They can think clearly, speak with confidence, able to focus on the task they were given and able to achieve their goals with a more determine mind. Along with more earned income, you can include money that is saved on medications, physicians fees, testing and other procedures. Healthy people are also more likely to be promoted at work to positions with higher salaries, thus they are easily become the senior management at a higher status.

Symptoms of Poor Blood Circulation

Once your brain stops receiving the amount of oxygen it needs to properly function, you could experience brain hypoxia. Symptoms of this brain hypoxia include memory loss, difficulty concentrating, loss of motor skills or movement of your body, and seizures. You are also at risk for a stroke.

Another indicator of poor circulation is a pale, sallow look to the skin. Someone with poor circulation will appear sickly, with a lack of healthy color in their face. This is due to the lack of blood flow to the capillaries under the skin. In addition to the lack of healthy color to the face, there is also an early onset of wrinkles and sagging skin. The premature aging of skin is just one of the visual symptoms of poor circulation. Smoking can contribute to poor circulation and premature aging of the skin. Contributing to a poor aesthetic could also be a lack of exercise, poor diet, poor skin care (try dry brushing), and a diet high in sodium.

Another visual symptom is varicose veins. Varicose veins have been plaguing more than just your Aunt Myrtle since humans began to walk upright. The veins most commonly affected are those in your lower extremities. They are caused by the failure of the valves in the veins that prevent blood from flowing backward into the vein. The fluid collects and creates bulging, often painful, protruding vessels. Your physician may recommend treatments ranging from lifestyle changes to surgery to resolve and prevent varicose veins. The lifestyle changes all focus around improving blood circulation, including losing weight.

Hair loss is another symptom those with poor circulation may experience. Hair follicles become deprived of required oxygen and nutrients to sustain healthy hair growth, causing the hair follicle to die off. Males who were diagnosed with male pattern baldness had a scalp blood flow three times lower than males with full heads of hair. You can stimulate more hair growth or prevent more hair loss, by increasing blood flow a few different ways. Scalp massage (using your hands or another's hands) not only increases blood flow but also reduces stress and tension that additionally can cause hair loss. Brushing your hair twice a day with a bristle brush will also stimulate and bring more blood flow to the scalp.

You can add weight gain and obesity to the list as well. This automatically puts you at risk for diabetes, hypertension, and heart disease. This is a hefty group of ailments to add to the mix! This could mean a lifetime of medicines, heart attacks, and expensive hospitalizations. Hypertension can also cause kidney failure as a result of damage to the arteries around the kidneys, as well as loss of vision.

You may also notice that your hands and feet are often cold or tingly in winter, sometimes even experiencing numbness, based on the severity of the blood flow restriction. Female is more likely to have cold feet than male as male generally has better blood circulation than female. That is why in generally speaking, middle age woman tends to get sick easier than middle age man.

Energy levels are greatly affected as well. Experiencing lethargy and shortness of breath is common in people who suffer from poor circulation. No matter how much they sleep, they just feel tired during the day. If you don't have the energy inside your body, how do you do a proper job at work? Lethargy will get you no where near your promotion or higher salary. Moreover, the impact on how they are able to enjoy their life is measurable, affecting daily activities from trips to the grocery store, family outings, and sex life.

With symptoms like these mounting, a person could fall victim to depression very easily. Dealing with multiple maladies, a decline in physical appearance, and not able to perform in life at full capacity, will eventually take a toll on mental health. As you look at the mirror and see an unhealthy appearance, you feel more depress and it will affect your health even more, and you are going in a vicious cycle. If you do not treat yourself right, at some point, you might feel so afraid that you do not look at the mirror anymore. The decline in physical appearance is an indirect symptom of the effects of poor circulation. Tending to your declining mental health along with other mounting health conditions will result in more money spent on medications and doctor visits. There is also the possibility of forever altering your brain chemistry with anti-depressants so that you may depend on the medications for life.

If you're not exercising or maintaining good blood circulation, you can expect more frequent visits to the doctor. Why spend money and time on doctors for your weak body while you can just spend time on exercise for your strong body? The money you could be spending on a new bicycle to ride or a gym membership ends up being spent on the health issues you have developed. This doesn't include the time missed from work, where you could put yourself at risk of being let go. No matter how hard you work, if you look weak and pale, your boss will never promote you in higher position. Even if you are a manager which lead a team of staff, your team just won't look up to you and follow your order. Please remember, people always look up to leader with strong characteristics with strong physical body. Even though many people dislike Donald Trump, he is able to demonstrate his power with his strong characteristics as a President of United States. But just imagine would he be the President if he looks sick and in need of medical supply? The answer certainly is "No". Therefore, guard your body well as your first priority, if your immune system is compromised, you must do something about this before your health declines even further! Prevention is better than cure!

Adequate sleep each night is paramount to support a healthy body and mind. Sleep apnea, insomnia, and three times the likelihood of developing hypertension are all possibilities that can happen to a person when they are sleep deprived. Poor blood circulation directly effects quality and length of sleep time and can result in any one of the mentioned sleep conditions.

How to Improve Blood Circulation

Now that you have more in-depth knowledge of the lengthy list of physical symptoms of poor blood circulation, it's time to learn different ways to increase your blood flow to improve your health and youthful appearance well into later life.

Many of the simple treatments involve the use of heat. Vessels expand upon exposure to heat, increasing blood circulation in the general area. Here are some simple, yet effective ways of treating and avoiding poor blood circulation:

<u>Vitamin C</u>

- Eat foods high in Vitamin C. It is a natural blood thinner, which allows the blood to flow more unrestricted and easily through your veins and capillaries. Vitamin C also promotes the production of collagen for glowing, youthful skin, and boosts immunity. Foods with a naturally high Vitamin C content include citrus fruits, strawberries, red bell peppers, pineapple (more Vitamin C than an orange!), kiwi, guava, brussels sprouts, kohlrabi, papaya, and kale. A simple change in diet can start improving your circulation before the day is over today! Consuming more fruits and vegetables high in Vitamin C will also deliver weight loss results, an added bonus of a healthy diet change.

Omega 3 Fatty Acids

- Eat foods high in Omega 3 fatty acids. These essential fatty acids support the cardiovascular system. Our bodies do not produce Omega 3 fatty acids on their own and they thus must be obtained through foods we consume. Foods high in Omega3 include Salmon and other fatty fishes, flaxseed oil, chia seeds, tofu, spinach, grass-fed beef, avocados, and navy beans. There are many resources with more extensive lists of food items rich in Omega 3 fatty acids. These fatty acids block multiple inflammation pathways in your cells and play a part in helping with blood clotting. Omega 3 fatty acids also help regulate our heart rhythm. Krill oil is a recommended supplement over fish oil because it is easier to absorb due to its attachment to phospholipids. There is less belching associated with krill oil than there was reported as common with fish oil. Omega 3 can be found in foods such as hemp, chia seeds, flaxseed, and a few others, but none of these foods contain DHA and EPA, that aids in fighting mental and physical diseases.

Supplements

- Take supplements on a regular basis. If you are an on-the-go person and you find it a challenge to prepare and include all the healthy food you should in your diet, supplements can offer a secondary source of essential vitamins and minerals. An alternative to costly medications, supplements are an affordable way to help support proper blood circulation. Plant sterols aid in the elimination of cholesterol consumed in your diet. But please do not overdose. Overdose of any supplements or medicine will damage your liver permanently. As the liver is a vital organ that plays a main role in detoxification, protein synthesis, glycogen storage and decomposition of red cells, so please do not overdose. I said this twice because some people worry about their health so much that they overdose and they died because of cirrhosis (dysfunction of liver due to long term damage).

Lycopene

- Lycopene has strong antioxidant properties. The function of antioxidants is to prevent and stop cell damage by inhibiting the oxidation of cells. Lycopene is found to reduce the risk factor of a heart attack or stroke by 3x's vs.

people who had lower levels of lycopene in their systems. Hawthorn extract causes vascular dilation and in turn, better blood circulation. In recent studies, regular use of hawthorn extract over at least 15 weeks reduced blood pressure.

Resveratrol

- Resveratrol is a powerful antioxidant found in many fruits and vegetables, but taking a supplement to get the maximum benefit of enhanced cardiac function may be easier for you. Bee pollen is a widely-used supplement containing rutin that works by strengthening your blood vessels and prevents the buildup of white blood cells in your arteries. It also aids in preventing blood clots that could alternatively end up causing a cardiac event or stroke.

Heat Your Body

- Use heat. Heat expands your blood vessels. This can include hot showers, baths, saunas, hot tubs, infrared light, and heating pads. None of these tools need to be exceedingly hot. A small increase in temperature will cause your blood vessels to expand. That's why Chinese love having saunas while Japanese love having a hot spring.

Both saunas and hot spring has the same principal to provide better blood circulation to people. A natural hot spring is even better for your skin because the mineral in the water has great benefits to your skin as the mineral can be easily absorbed by your skin in heated water. Japanese girls have smooth skin because they love hot spring. Infrared light effectively improves blood circulation as much as exercise, and aids in pain relief and healing of wounds and injuries. It is widely used in sports medicine due to the efficiency and speed at which it gets players back on the field. Saunas are also a treatment proven to have coronary benefits, normalizing blood pressure, and increasing blood flow to your muscles. A sauna session just one time to two times a week can make vast improvements in blood circulation. You may want to avoid saunas if you have existing blood pressure issues. Applying a heating pad to the tops of your feet. Once your blood has traveled to the bottom of your extremities, it has to fight gravity to get back up to your heart again. If your vessels are constricted, this makes the task even more difficult. If you suffer from continually cold feet and hands, applying a heating pad to the top of your feet where your skin is thin and many large veins are present will expand the vessels and make the process of delivering blood back up to the heart easier for your body.

Heat Your Feet

- Heat your feet everyday! Making sure you keep your feet warm increases peripheral blood flow. Having cold feet could be a result of cold weather, cold floors in your home, a symptom of a circulation restrictive health condition such as Raynaud's disease or diabetes. In Chinese, they think that the benefits of put your feet in hot water are similar to eating expensive food with high nutrition value. Keeping your feet warm can be used as a preventative measure to ensure better blood circulation on a regular basis, or as a counteractive measure, once coldness has set in. You do not need to spend a lot of money of supplements and food if your budget is limited, heating your feet don't cost much. Some of the methods of keeping your feet warm include; using your own metabolic rate to warm up your feet while they are covered in very warm socks or down slippers, soaking your feet in a warm pot of water, wrap them with a heating pad. Heating pad is useful because you can control and keep consistent heat on your feet for any length of time, applying a hot water bottle, or wrapping your feet and lower extremities in an electric blanket. The temperature of your feet affects your whole body, causing vessel constriction as cooler blood is circulated. Studies have shown that having chronically cold feet can also increase your risk of catching a cold because of vessel constriction in the nose, which decreases the amount of white blood vessels available to fight off a common cold.

Exercise

- Doing exercise regularly. Just 30 minutes a day of exercise will produce profound positive changes within your body. There are many different forms of exercise that you can do, even for those who have limited physical abilities. Getting enough exercise does not have to cost any money. Outside of the typical gym membership, yoga classes, spinning classes and pilates, there are many other activities you can easily integrate into your daily routine. Throwing a football in the backyard with your kids, playing a couple of games of driveway basketball, going for a bike ride with your family or friends, or just a brisk walk around the block, can make noticeable changes in the way your circulation performs and how your body looks and feels. Athletes and soldiers usually have no problem with blood circulation as they do different kinds of exercise on a regular basis. Not only they have stronger muscles and body, but also they have better skin as the blood under their skin is kept flowing. Athletes have better motivation and usually have positive emotion and self-esteem. Higher level of self-esteem plays an important part of an individual's sex appeal. If impact exercises are out of your reach, stretching is a low-impact, easy way to improve circulation to your organs and muscles. This can be done sitting in a chair, standing, lying in bed, or on the floor. You might try some free instructional videos on the internet, or ask what stretches your physician recommends to avoid injuring yourself.

Sleep At The Right Time

- Getting enough exercise also contributes to deeper, longer sleep. Adults should get 7 to 9 hours of sleep each night to achieve maximum benefits, including a period of REM sleep. Sleep deprivation increases blood pressure. Studies have shown that neural cardiovascular control is negatively impacted when subjects did not get enough sleep. While you sleep, your body goes to work repairing blood vessels, your brain and other vital tissues that support your cardiovascular health. Going to bed earlier and ditching "night owl" habits has an even greater impact. Lack of sleep also causes stress. Daily tasks and otherwise easier-to-handle life events seem more difficult to cope with, elevating blood pressure. Adequate sleep supports an important homeostatic function of regulating blood pressure. You may want to look into why your quality of sleep is poor, and implement new sleeping positions and tools to improve your sleep each night. Make sure your neck is not craned and that other body parts are not bent or distorted in a way that may cut off blood circulation. Choosing a blood circulation friendly position to fall asleep in each night can help with a more restful sleep. Consider a new mattress and pillows. It has been found that sleeping on your side is the recommended sleep position. There are many benefits to side-sleeping, two of which are flushing harmful waste from your body via the glymphatic systems, and increasing blood flow to your heart. If you have exhausted all of these options and still have trouble sleeping, try a little more exercise during the day, take a few deep breathe at night in your bed or consult with your physician.

<u>Drink Water To Cleanse Your Body</u>

- Drink more water. Not just any water, but hot or warm water in the morning. Many of us enjoy a crisp glass of ice cold water, but if you are trying to increase your blood circulation, it could be counter-productive. Warm water acts in the same ways as the other heat methods, expanding your blood vessels in your digestive tract and aids in the digestion process, better eliminating fats from your meals. This is a beneficial effect vs. cold water which causes the fat to solidify. Just like bacon grease in the pan. Once it cools off, it is solid and white and harder to eliminate from your intestines. Adding fresh squeezed lemon to the water for taste is a healthy way to add some flavor, in addition to turning your glass of warm water into its own super drink. Fresh lemon contains natural enzymes that assist your liver in getting rid of toxins. Rich in flavonoids that increase blood flow circulation, they also pack a punch of Vitamin C. At the very least, drink one glass of warm water each morning, but feel free to add a few more glasses throughout the day and night or with meals to get the most out of this circulation boosting method.

Vitamin D

- Soak up the sun! Vitamin D plays a critical role in healthy vasculature. Hypovitaminosis D, or vitamin D deficiency, The muscles in your heart need calcitriol to maintain and build healthy tissues, and vitamin D is converted into calcitriol through a special process. Not only is vitamin D a nutrient, it is also a hormone that plays many important roles in our bodies and circulatory health. Ways to provide your body with vitamin D are direct exposure to sunlight and supplements. Exposing your skin directly to sunlight, which contains the UVB rays that prompt the production of vitamin D in our bodies. There are limited foods that contain vitamin D naturally, so it is easy to become deficient. In order to produce sufficient vitamin D naturally, you need only expose your skin to direct sunlight for about 15 minutes. Getting a sunburn or prolonged sun exposure will not produce more vitamin D. The process happens quickly within your body. Your body can produce between 10,000 and 25,000 IU (International Units) of vitamin D in that short amount of time. If you have darker skin, you may require a few extra minutes of sun exposure than those with pale skin. If you choose to go the supplement route, there are many good quality brands and types to choose from.

There are several websites dedicated to testing and providing information on different brands of vitamin D, including which ones to avoid that may contain lead and other harmful elements like mercury, arsenic, and cadmium. Their studies show that the pill type did not affect the quality of the supplement, so choosing between a gelcap, tablet, and capsule makes no difference. Consult with your health care professional on your specific dosing needs. Most adults should not exceed 4,000 IU without a doctor's recommendation.

Feel Happy and Laugh More

- Laugh more! Studies have shown that after 15 minutes of viewing a TV show that induced laughter, 70% of the test subjects showed increased cardiovascular blood flow. Laughter produced the same effect as physical exercise without any of the pain and soreness. It also reduces the amount of the stress hormone cortisol. This could be one of the easiest ways to lower your blood pressure and prevent diabetes. People who laughed after eating a meal also had lower blood glucose levels than those who did not laugh. Laughter lifts the spirits and reduces overall stress.

Consider this one of the easiest ways to improve your circulation.

Foot Reflexology / Foot Massage

- Try foot massage. Reflexology technically is not "massage" in its practical form. It is a reflex therapy. Foot reflexology is greatly applied in Chinese to cure disease as it would unclog your blood stream in variety of organs. It uses the application of pressure to different reflex points on the body, specifically the feet, head, hands, and ears. It is generally safe, and promotes a state of relaxation and increased blood flow to various parts of the body by applying pressure to the specific points on the bottom of your foot. Each point of your feet related to certain part of your body, if you feel pain when having foot reflexology, it means that you have some problems with certain part of your body and more reflex therapy is required to cure that part of your body. It is proven to aid in the increase of certain body functions by clearing neural pathways. Reflexology helps to increase circulation and deliver more adequate levels of blood and oxygen to your entire body, enabling your body to heal faster and return to more normal metabolic processes.

Swedish Massage

- Swedish massage. A full body massage, specifically the Swedish massage, a few times a week lowers blood pressure more than if you were to just relax for that same amount of time. Swedish massage increases circulation without putting undue strain on the heart. It also aids in cleansing the glands and releasing toxins. Swedish massage applies pressure down deep to the muscles, pressing against other deeper muscles and bones, and rubbing in the direction that the blood flows to the heart (effleurage).

Dry Brushing

- Dry brushing your skin uses a handheld bristle brush in gentle strokes all over your skin to stimulate blood flow, remove dead cells, and move toxins through the lymphatic system. Dry brushing also makes your skin vibrant with a healthy glow because dead cells are removed, exposing new, healthy skin cells. Typically, you would dry brush your whole body just before you shower, so you can rinse off the loosened dead skin cells. Try dry brushing once a day as a simple way to increase blood flow circulation to your skin.

The DONT'S! Things to avoid that reduce blood circulation

DON'T: <u>Consume Sugary Drinks, Caffeine, Or Alcohol.</u>
Even adding 1 sugary drink to your daily intake can contribute to weight gain and a 25% greater risk of developing type II diabetes. Caffeine is a stimulant that increases your blood pressure. It has been shown to decrease cerebral blood flow by 27%! If you are a regular caffeine beverage drinker and cut out caffeine, you will have increased cerebral blood flow within 30 hours of your last beverage. A very simple change. While consuming 1 alcoholic beverage per day (A glass of wine, for example) can help maintain healthy circulation, drinking alcohol in excess can negatively affect the cells of endothelium and smooth muscle, both of which work to control blood circulation. Alcohol consumption keeps these cells from working properly.

DON'T: <u>Avoid Caffeinated Teas Such As Green Tea, Black Tea, and Matcha</u>
Though rich in antioxidants, these drinks contain caffeine. I have already covered the negative effects of caffeine on your circulatory

30

system. Opt for a caffeine free version, although finding one at a supplement dispensary that has no caffeine may prove to be a challenge. Daily flaxseed oil capsules also reduce the chances of a heart attack. There are many knowledgeable specialists that can help walk you through the best supplement options for your situation and circulation challenges. The quality of supplements plays a huge role in their performance. Research the origin and purity of the different brands you come across; otherwise, you may just be spending money on old, dead plants in a pill form that offer no nutrition, are hard for your body to break down, and have limited bioavailability.

DON'T: <u>Go Long Periods Of Time Being Stationary</u>

A sedentary lifestyle will first and foremost become your worst enemy in damaging your circulatory system. One in ten cases of heart disease is caused by a lack of exercise. You also increase your risk of developing diabetes and cancer. Lack of exercise causes almost as many deaths as smoking! On days that you do not exercise, your blood pressure increases. After 2 weeks of no exercise, changes to your blood vessels occur. It will take about another week of exercise to reverse these changes and bring your vessels back to a healthy, higher functioning state. When you exercise, your glucose levels remain higher because your muscles and tissues use the sugars you consume for energy. Without regular exercise, your glucose levels will continue to increase. This is particularly dangerous if you have existing diabetes, but can also prime you for developing the dangerous health condition.

DON'T: <u>Walk Around Outside On Cold Days, Or On Cold Floors Inside With Bare Feet Or Flimsy Shoes</u>

Keeping your feet warm is one of the easiest and effective methods you can practice easily on a regular basis to avoid reducing your overall body temperature and restricting peripheral blood flow, and increasing your susceptibility of catching a cold due to the reduction of available white blood cells within your nose that fight off the virus.

DON'T: <u>Smoke!</u>

The dangers and consequences of smoking are endless. I could write an entire other book on the negative effects of smoking on the body. But if you are specifically worried about improving your blood circulation, this would be one of the first things to cut out of your life. Nicotine itself has been shown to grow new blood vessels within our existing vessels, hardening our arteries and promoting more clogging. Smoking affects every vessel in your body. Smoking also causes our brain to go into "fight or flight" mode, triggering the release of stored fats and sugars for 'emergency' situations and immediate use for energy, into your blood stream. This is especially detrimental to anyone with diabetes because it triggers a spike in glucose levels every time you smoke! This is also why smoking curbs your appetite and causes you to crave another cigarette soon after, because you are essentially skipping meals and the release of the stored fats and sugars are "feeding" you. Smoking will prematurely age your skin. There is no reversing aged skin. The only way to keep your youthful look is by preventative care, which includes **stopping smoking.**

DON'T: <u>Consume high sodium foods.</u>

This works doubly well when you couple lowering your sodium intake with adding the foods that increase blood flow to your diet. Sodium causes hardening of your arteries, which leads to high blood pressure. Reducing sodium in your diet takes a little more than not putting salt on your food. You need to look at the nutritional information of your food *before* you add salt, so you know exactly what you are consuming. If you have a health condition such as high blood pressure, the recommended daily amount of sodium intake is 1,500mg per day. If you are relatively healthy, the average person is recommended to stay at or below

33

2,300mg per day. Sodium plays an important role in our bodies muscle and nerve function and regulation of blood pressure, so eliminating all sodium from your diet is not recommended and can end up causing more severe problems than just poor circulation!

Conclusion

In conclusion, improving your blood circulation can be done easily by making just a few small life changes. From keeping your feet warm to brushing your scalp, dry brushing your skin to going for a walk 30 minutes a day, all of the recommendations are attainable in some way, by every person.

If you have questions or difficulties incorporating the recommended foods (the mentioned beneficial foods are a limited list of what is actually available. Do your research!) into your diet, the internet has an expansive library of affordable, easy recipes to follow.

You may not feel immediate effects of some of the methods. Although some of these methods are effective right away, some of them will *prevent* undesirable conditions and symptoms down the road. Combining as many suggested methods as possible will help ensure you maintain, or improve your blood circulation.

If you are unsure of dosages or you suffer from complicated health issues, you may want to be monitored under a physician's care so that you can implement these methods in the safest way for you.

Thanks For Reading!

If you interest in any other topics, email me at

alan_toast@hotmail.com